Mastery of Obesity

Know the Effects of Weight Gain and Healthy Habits to Beat Body Fat

By

Dorothy J. Casey

TABLE OF CONTENTS

Introduction

Contrary to popular belief, America does not have the greatest obesity rates in the world, but it routinely ranks in the top 20. (If you're curious, countries from Oceania often top the list, with Arabic countries also scoring high).

Why does America continue to rank first in the world in terms of obesity? It all comes down to a few things. One of the most significant is, of course, the average American diet. Consider Japan, a country that constantly ranks around the bottom of the obesity scale. The traditional Japanese diet is high in seafood and vegetables, with little sugar or fat. Perhaps more crucially, serving portions are maintained to a minimum. America has had decades of incredible agricultural richness, which has encouraged us to go big or go home in terms of servings. More food consumption equals more weight gain.

But, there are more subtle explanations behind America's obesity epidemic. Much of how we work and live is geared to make us acquire weight, even if unintentionally.

Consider American cities. Many American communities are intended to be exclusively accessible by car. A lack of daily walking opportunities can contribute to weight gain.

Consider the occupations we do these days, you are less likely to go outside for work or even move around the workplace. Everything we require is conveniently located at a single computer, which is frequently located in our homes.

There's no compelling reason to leave our cozy workspace chairs and part of it must be attributed to laziness. Obesity has been in America for a long time now, we have been residing in for so long, we've simply ignored the obesity pandemic. It was accepted as a feature of the American landscape.

Obesity could have been reduced to a punchline jokes at the cost of America, but it's not funny.

Greater BMIs have a variety of negative implications on your overall health, such as an increased risk of high blood pressure high blood pressure, diabetes, heart disease, gallbladder disease, arthritis, sleep apnea, mental disorders, and even cancer.

All of these conditions can be treated with medicine. Therefore, the ideal solution is simply to never come across them at all. That entails dealing with your excessive BMI directly to reduce the severity of these dangers.

Obesity prevents you from doing the things you enjoy, such as spending time with family and friends, and it makes you unhappy less confident in yourself, which progressively causes you to feel depressed, and sometimes in your search for a solution, it's possible that you'll spend a fortune.

This book has a few pages that are jam-packed with obesity information that you must be aware of as well as how to overcome it.

CHAPTER 1
The definition of obesity

Obesity is a medical disorder that arises when a person is overweight. Excess weight or body fat may jeopardize their health.

A doctor will usually recommend that a person be diagnosed with obesity if they have an elevated body mass index (BMI).

Obesity, often known as corpulence or fatness, is an excess of body fat.

Body fat accumulation, mainly induced by consuming more calories than the body can use. Excess calories are subsequently stored as fat, or adipose tissue.

Overweight, if moderate, is not always harmful, especially in muscular or large-boned people individuals.

What exactly is BMI?

BMI is a metric that doctors use to determine whether or not a patient is overweight.

A person's weight is adequate for their age, gender, and height. It adds up a person's weight in kilograms divided by the square of their height in meters.

Obesity measurement using BMI

A BMI of 25 to 29.9 suggests that a person is overweight. If a person is obese, they have a BMI of 30 or higher.

Other indicators include a person's waist-to-hip ratio, waist-to-height ratio, and the amount and distribution of fat.

The amount of fat they have also plays a role in deciding how healthy their weight is.

CHAPTER 2
Factors that leads to obesity

Obesity is a complex disease that happens when an individual's weight exceeds what is deemed healthy for his or her height. Obesity can be seen in both children and adults. Several causes can contribute to excessive weight gain, and some of these aspects will be examined:

- Diet
- Physical exercise
- Hereditary
- Diseases
- Pharmaceuticals
- Age and other factors that will be mentioned.

DIET

If you consume a lot of energy, especially from high fat and high sugar foods, and do not expend all of it through physical exercise, a lot of it will be stored as fat in your body.

Consuming high amount of calories

Food's energy content is measured in units called calories. The average physically active male requires about 2,500 calories a day to keep a healthy weight, and the average physically active person requires approximately 2,000 calories. A day's worth of calories. This number of calories may appear to be excessive, yet it is not.

If you eat particular foods, it is simple to obtain that amount of calories. For instance, eating a huge takeaway hamburger, fries, and a single milkshake can contain up to 1,500 calories.

Furthermore, many people do not meet the recommended levels of physical exercise for adults, so Excess calories consumed are stored as fat in the body.

Obesity-creating eating habits

- **Eating a lot of processed or fast food** - this is food high in fat and sugar.

- **Too much alcohol consumption** - alcohol contains a lot of calories. Individuals can consume a lot of calories without getting fat or feeling full, particularly calories from alcohol, might be detrimental contribute to severe weight gain.

- **Eating out frequently** - restaurant meals may contain allergens.

- **Drinking too many sugary drinks**-. Some high-calorie beverages, such as sugared soft drinks, can also contribute to weight gain.

- **Comfort eating** - some people may comfort eat as a result of many other factors affecting their lives, such as low self-esteem or depression. Changes in society have also made it more difficult to maintain a healthy diet. High-calorie food has grown more affordable and easy, and it is widely sold and pushed.

PHYSICAL EXERCISE

Another key factor associated with obesity is a lack of physical activity. Many people work jobs that require them to sit at a desk for the majority of the day. People also drive their cars instead of walking or cycling. Many people watch TV, surf the internet, or play computer games to unwind, and they rarely exercise on a regular basis.

If you are not physically active enough, you will not use the energy provided by the food you eat, and any excess energy will be stored as fat by the body.

HEREDITARY

Certain genes have been linked to fat and overweight. Genes can influence how and where fat is stored and dispersed in some people. Genetics may also influence how efficiently your body transforms food into energy, how your body regulates your hunger, and how efficiently your body burns calories during exercise. Obesity is often passed down to individuals in families. This isn't just because they share genes. Family members also have similar food and physical activity patterns.

Some genetic features inherited from your parents, such as a voracious appetite, may make reducing weight more difficult, but not impossible.

DISEASES AND PHARMACEUTICAL

Diseases

A few diseases that might lead to excess weight are given below.

- **Hypothyroidism** is a thyroid disorder. This is a condition in which the thyroid gland, located in the neck, generates excessive amounts of thyroid hormone.

Thyroid hormone is in short supply that affects our metabolic rate. As a result, the metabolism is often slowed, resulting in weight gain. If your doctor suspects that you have thyroid illness, they may check your hormone levels with blood testing.

- **Cushing's syndrome** this situation occurs when the adrenal glands (located on top of each kidney) overproduce a steroid hormone.

Cortisol is a hormone. Among other things, it causes fat to accumulate in prominent areas such as the face and upper arms, back, as well as the abdomen.

Obesity in some persons can be linked to a medical condition, such as Prader-Willi syndrome or Cushing syndrome as well as other circumstances. Medical issues, such as arthritis, can also cause a decrease in exercise, which can lead to weight gain. There are also inherited conditions and other brain illnesses that might lead to weight gain.

PHARMACEUTICALS

Some pharmaceuticals, most notably steroids, as well as certain antidepressants, antipsychotics, hypertension medicines, and seizure meds can also produce weight gain or hindering weight decrease

AGE

Obesity can strike at any age, including children. But Hormonal changes and a less active lifestyle as you age Increase your chances of being obese. Also, the amount of muscle in your body tends to decline with age. Lower muscle mass generally leads to a decrease in metabolism. These modifications also cut calorie requirements and can make losing weight more difficult. If you do not consciously limit what you eat and become more active, you will gain weight.
If you are physically active as you age, you will most certainly acquire weight.

OTHER FACTORS

Pregnancy weight increase is frequent. Some women find it difficult to reduce this weight after having children. Excessive weight gain could be a factor in obesity among women.

Smoking cessation. Stopping smoking is frequently related with weight gain. And for some, it may cause the person gain too much weight that would lead to obesity. This frequently occurs when people use food to cope with quitting smoking. In the long run, however, quitting smoking is still a better health choice than smoking. Your doctor can assist you in avoiding weight gain after stopping smoking.

Inadequate sleep. Getting too little or too much sleep might induce hormonal changes, increase your appetite. You may also develop appetite for foods with high calories and carbohydrates that can cause obesity.

Getting stressed out. There are numerous extrinsic influences that influence mood and behavior. Obesity may be influenced by one's level of happiness. Humans frequently when faced with a stressful scenario, eat extra high-calorie foods.

The microbiome. What influences your gut bacteria is what you consume, which might lead to weight gain or trouble decreasing weight. Even if you have one or more of these risk factors, you are not doomed to develop obesity.

The majority of risk factors can be mitigated by nutrition, physical activity and exercise, as well as behavioral modifications which will be discussed in chapter 5

CHAPTER 3
Obesity risk factor

Obesity and overweight may increase your chance of some health problems as well as certain emotional and social problems.

Diabetes mellitus type 2

Type 2 diabetes is a condition that develops when your blood glucose, also known as blood sugar, is abnormally high. Around 8 out of 10 patients with type 2 diabetes are overweight or obese. High blood glucose levels cause difficulties such as heart disease, stroke, renal disease, vision problems, nerve damage, and other health issues over time.

If you are at risk for type 2 diabetes, decreasing 5 to 7% of your body weight and engaging in regular physical activity may help you avoid or postpone the beginning of the disease.

High blood pressure

High blood pressure, often known as hypertension, is a disorder in which blood rushes more forcefully through your blood vessels than is usual. High blood pressure can cause heart strain, blood vessel damage, and an increased risk of heart attack, stroke, renal illness, and death.

Cardiovascular disease

Heart disease refers to a variety of issues that can affect your heart. You should avoid smoking if you have heart disease may suffer from a heart attack, heart failure, or a sudden cardiac arrest death, angina, or an irregular heart rhythm are all possibilities. High blood pressure, abnormal blood levels, high blood glucose levels and saturated fats may increase your risk of heart disease. Blood fats, commonly known as blood lipids, HDL cholesterol, LDL cholesterol, and

Triglycerides are types of blood fat.

Reducing 5 to 10% of your body weight may reduce your risk factors for acquiring heart disease. If you weigh 200 pounds,

This means you could lose as little as 10 pounds weight. Weight loss of weight may lower blood pressure, cholesterol levels, and the flow of blood.

Stroke

A stroke is a disorder in which the blood supply to your brain is disrupted.

Because of a blockage or the breaking of a blood artery in your brain or neck. A stroke can cause brain tissue damage and render you unable to talk or move certain areas of your body. Elevated blood pressure is the cause. Strokes are the most common cause of death.

Sleep apnea

Sleep apnea is a prevalent disorder in which you do not breathe regularly while sleeping. For brief periods of time, you may cease breathing entirely. Sleep Apnea that has not been treated may increase your risk of developing other health issues, such as **type 2 diabetes** and **heart disease.**

Metabolic Syndrome

Metabolic syndrome is a collection of illnesses that increases your risk of heart disease, diabetes, and stroke. These circumstances are

- blood pressure that is too high (High blood pressure)
- high levels of blood glucose
- immoderate amounts of triglycerides in your blood
- low HDL cholesterol (the "good" cholesterol) levels in your blood
- excessive fat around the waist

Fatty liver disorders

Are ailments that occur when fat accumulates in the liver. Nonalcoholic fatty liver disease (NAFLD) and

Nonalcoholic steatohepatitis (NASH) are the two types of fatty liver disorder. Fatty liver disease can result in severe liver damage, cirrhosis, or even liver failure are all possibilities.

Osteoarthritis

Osteoarthritis is a common, long-term health issue that causes pain, swelling, and decreased motion in your joints.

Joints being overweight or obese may increase your risk of developing osteoarthritis by putting extra strain on your joints and cartilage.

Gallbladder problems

Obesity and being overweight may increase your risk of Gallbladder illnesses, such as gallstones and cholecystitis can occur. Gallstones are caused by imbalances in the chemicals that make up bile. Gallstones can develop if the bile contains an excessive amount of cholesterol.

Several types of cancer

Cancer NIH external link is a collection of connected diseases. Some of the body's cells begin to divide uncontrollably and spread into surrounding tissues in all types of cancer. Obesity and overweight may increase your risk of acquiring some types of cancer NIH external link.

Kidney failure

Kidney disease indicates that your kidneys have been damaged and are unable to filter blood as effectively as they should. Obesity increases the most common risk factors for diabetes and high blood pressure, Promote renal disease and hasten its progression.

 Obesity may be harmful even if you do not have diabetes or high blood pressure.

Pregnancy complications

Obesity and overweight increase the risk of health complications. This is something that can happen during pregnancy. Overweight or obese pregnant women may have a higher risk of miscarriage acquiring gestational diabetes experiencing preeclampsia—high blood pressure during pregnancy, which can lead to serious health problems , If left untreated, this can cause complications for both the mother and the infant requiring a cesarean section NIH external link, or C-section and hence requiring longer to recover following childbirth.

CHAPTER 4
Signs of obesity

Early indications of obesity

The most noticeable obesity symptoms and indicators are excess body fat and weight gain. Other signs and symptoms of obesity include:

> - Difficulty sleeping (daytime drowsiness, sleep apnea) Joint pain
> - Excessive sweating
> - Shortness of breath
> - Infections in the skin folds
> - Intolerance to heat Fatigue
> - Depression
> - Irregular menstrual cycles
> - Late indication of obesity

Late indications of obesity

Often occur due to the magnitude of weight gain; as a result, a person may notice the following:

> - In the legs, there is swelling and varicose veins.
> - Acanthosis nigricans is a skin disorder that causes hyperpigmentation and hyperkeratosis in the armpits and skin folds.

- ➤ Stretch marks are caused by the skin's elastic fibers rupturing.
- ➤ Blood pressure that is too high.
- ➤ A BMI of more than 30 kg/m2 is considered obese.
- ➤ Waist circumference: greater than 88 cm in women and greater than 94 cm in males.

BMI is often used by doctors to define obesity. The BMI compares the bodily weight to the body surface area. Doctors use the BMI to evaluate if a person is healthy, overweight, or obese.

Obesity is classified into classes by doctors based on its severity.

1. **Class I** obesity is defined as having a BMI ranging from 30 to 34.9 kg/m2.

2. **Class II** obesity is defined as having a BMI ranging from 35 to 39.9 kg/m2.

3. **Class III** obesity, commonly known as morbid obesity, occurs when a person begins to experience obesity-related health problems. Class III BMI is 40 kg/m2 and above.

However, BMI has several restrictions, such as in the case of sportsmen and bodybuilders, who have increased muscle mass.

Muscles outnumber fat. They may also have a high BMI but a low body mass index Fat on the body.

CHAPTER 5
Conquering obesity

1. Healthy Eating
Fruits

- Whether the fruits are served fresh, frozen, or canned, they are all brilliant options.

- Try mango with other fruits other than apples and bananas pineapple or kiwi.

- When fresh fruit is not available consider using a frozen, canned, or dried variety. (Dried and canned fruit may contain additional sugars or syrups. Instead, select canned fruit that contains water or its own juice.)

Vegetables

- Use a herb like rosemary to add flavor to grilled or cooked veggies.

- Vegetables can also be sautéed (fried).With a small quantity of cooking spray, cook in a nonstick pan.

- For a quick side meal, utilize frozen or canned vegetables. Just microwave and serve.

- Choose canned vegetables that have no added salt, butter, or cream sauces.

(To add variation, every week, try a new veggie.)

Calcium-containing foods

Choose low-fat and fat-free yogurts without added sugars in addition to fat-free and low-fat milk. These are available.

It comes in a variety of flavors and makes an excellent dessert substitute.

Meats

- If your favorite dish asks for frying fish or breaded chicken, consider baking or grilling it instead.

- Try switching into dry beans for beef.

- With your friends, you can look for recipes on the internet and in publications with less calories you may be shocked to discover a new favorite recipe!

Foods of Solace

Even if your favorite foods are rich in calories, fat, or added sweets, you can still enjoy them. The key is to eat.

These should only be used once in a while.

Some general recommendations for comfort foods:

- **Do not consume them frequently.** If you regularly consume these items reduce your daily consumption to once a week or once a month.

- **Cut down on high-calorie meal.** If your favorite higher-calorie meal is a chocolate bar, eat it in lesser portions or only once.

- **Go for a lower-calorie version of meal.** Utilize low-calorie foods ingredients or make cuisine in a different way. As an example, if your macaroni and cheese recipe calls for whole milk try remaking it with nonfat milk, less butter, low-fat cheese, and fresh herbs instead of full-fat milk, butter, and cheese tomatoes and spinach. But keep in mind not to raise your portion size.

- **Fasting on alternate days**. Another method for reducing food consumption is intermittent fasting that is gaining popularity as a weight-loss technique and health advantages. One type is alternate-day fasting, a type of intermittent fasting that includes a "fast day" (eating only one-fourth of one's caloric needs) alternated with a "fed day," or a day with no restrictions. Only a few studies on intermittent fasting as a weight loss technique have been undertaken. They have no long-term data on safety and benefits of intermittent fasting for long-term weight loss maintenance.

2. Participate In Physical Exercises

The Ministry of Health and Social Care suggests that people engage in at least 150 minutes of moderate-intensity exercise every week, engage in aerobic activities such as cycling or rapid walking weekly. This does not have to be completed at once. Although it can be divided into smaller periods.
You could, for example, exercise for 30 minutes five days a week.

If you have obesity and are attempting to reduce weight, you may need to undertake more activity than this. It could be beneficial to begin carefully and progressively expand your weekly workout routine.

The two types of exercises to engage in:

Progressive: If your breathing and pulse rate are substantially faster while undertaking the physical activity but you can still carry on a conversation, it's definitely fairly intense. Here are several examples:

- Walking quickly (a 15-minute mile).
- Mild yard work (raking/bagging leaves or mowing the lawn).
- Minimal snow shoveling is required.
- Playing actively with children.
- Biking at a leisurely pace.

Energetic: Your heart rate has significantly increased and you are breathing too rapidly and too hard to hold a conversation.

It's most likely a difficult conversation. Examples include:

- Jogging or running.
- Swimming laps.
- Inline skating/rollerblading at a fast pace.

- Skiing on the cross-country course.
- Sports with the highest level of competition (football, basketball, or soccer). Rope jumping.

Conclusion

Obesity does not have a "quick fix." Weight loss programs and changing of diets require time and commitment, and they perform best when fully completed. The healthcare providers who are involved in your treatment should provide support and ideas on how to keep the weight loss that was accomplished.

Setting realistic objectives and regularly monitoring your weight as well as enlisting your friends and family in your endeavors to losing weight can also be beneficial.

Note that even a seemingly insignificant loss can have a significant impact.
It is possible to lose a significant amount of weight, such as 3% or more of your initial body weight, and maintain the body weight for the rest of your life, can reduce your chance of developing obesity-related problems such as diabetes and heart disease.

www.ingramcontent.com/pod-product-compliance
Lightning Source LLC
Chambersburg PA
CBHW061600250726
48657CB00021B/2440